DILL

MARIAN KIM

CONTENTS

1

PROPERTIES

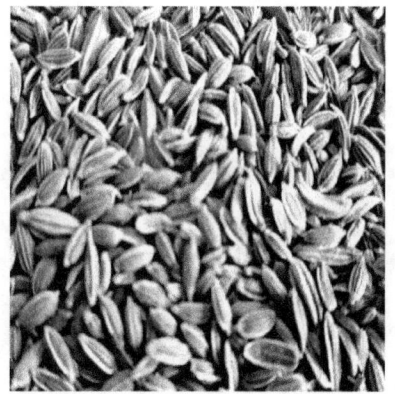

Scientific name: Anethum graveolens

Other names: Aneth, dillweed, dilly

Nutrients: Vitamin C, calcium, manganese, magnesium, fiber

Properties

Antiseptic (antibacterial, antifungal) properties

Abortifacient (can cause miscarriage) properties

Anticancer properties since it contains monoterpenes which limit the growth of cancer cells in the body.

Carminative (anti-flatulent) properties

Diuretic (increase urine production) properties

Galactogogue (increase breast milk) properties

Stomachic (stimulate digestion and relieve stomach pain) properties

Insect repellent properties

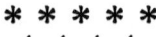

2

USES

Insomnia treatment

Dill has a calming effect which may be beneficial for managing insomnia.

Colic relief

Dill water is used to relieve colic in babies.

Flatulence treatment

Dill is used to relieve flatulence due to its carminative properties.

Upset stomach relief

Dill tea is used to soothe an upset stomach.

Diarrhea treatment

Dill is used to assist in the management of diarrhea due to its anti-microbial effects. It also soothes the intestines.

Anorexia treatment

Dill is used for loss of appetite.

Sore eye treatment

A dill compress can be used to reduce the inflammation of sore eyes. To make one steep dill seeds in boiling water for 2 minutes and dip a clean cloth in the tea. Apply the warm compress on the closed eyelids for 20 minutes.

Breast milk induction

Dill tea is used to increase breast milk production by nursing mothers.

Period induction

Dill tea is used to bring on menstrual periods in women who have late or scanty periods since its essential oils can regulate the menstrual cycle. It is also used for menstrual cramps.

Fever treatment

Dill is used to treat fever.

Coughs and colds treatment

Dill is used to reduce the symptoms of coughs and colds. It is also used for bronchitis.

Urinary tract disorders

Dill which has diuretic properties, is used for urinary tract disorders like painful or difficult urination.

Liver and gall bladder disorders

Dill is used for liver and gall bladder problems.

Halitosis treatment

Dill is used to manage halitosis (bad breath) since it freshens the breath. Its essential oils also have antimicrobial properties which can fight the microbes in the mouth.

Mouth ulcers treatment

Dill is used to reduce the pain and swelling of inflamed mouth and throat conditions.

Hemorrhoid treatment

Dill is used for hemorrhoids.

Genital ulcer treatment

Dill is used for genital ulcers.

Spasm relief

Dill is used to relieve spasms.

Hiccup relief

Dill is used to relieve hiccups.

Nerve pain relief

Dill is used to relieve nerve pain.

Skin lesion management

Dill poultices are used for skin lesions like cysts.

Infections

Dill is used for infections since it has antiseptic (antibacterial, antifungal) properties.

Insect repellent

Dill has insect repellent properties.

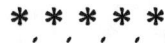

3

SAFETY PRECAUTIONS

1. Pregnant women should not use dill in medicinal amounts since it might cause miscarriages.

2. Dill can cause allergic reactions to persons who are allergic to plants in the carrot family like caraway, celery, coriander and fennel.

3. Fresh dill juice can make the skin become more sensitive to the sun. This can lead to increase risks for developing sunburns and skin cancer. Therefore light-skinned persons should apply sunscreen and wear protective clothing.

4. Dill can cause skin irritation when applied on the skin.

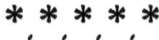

4

DRUG INTERACTIONS

1. Dill interacts with lithium since it has a diuretic effect in the body. It might therefore reduce the excretion of lithium from the body and increase lithium side effects.

* * * * *

5

COOKING TIPS

Flavor: Fresh

Goes well with: Salads e.g. tuna salad, egg dishes e.g. omelets, dressings e.g. yogurt dressing, poultry e.g. chicken, vegetables e.g. cucumbers, carrots, cabbage and potatoes, beets, tomatoes and potatoes, legumes e.g. green beans, seafood, vinegars, dips e.g. yogurt dips, rice, fish especially grilled

Can be substituted with: Caraway, basil

Tips: Can be added to food just before serving.

* * * * *

6

HERBAL RECIPES

Dill Tea

Equipment

Kettle

Tea cup

***

Ingredients

1 teaspoon of finely crushed or minced dill

1 cup of boiling water

Honey to taste (optional)

***

Instructions

1. Put the dill in a tea cup, add the boiling water and let it steep while covered for 10 -15 minutes.

2. Add honey (if using) to suit your taste before drinking.

*****

Dill Syrup

Equipment

Saucepan

Jar with airtight lid

***

Ingredients

1 quart (1000 ml) filtered water

1 cup dried dill or 3 cups fresh dill

1 cup honey

***

Instructions

1. Place the water and dill in a saucepan and bring to a boil.

2. Reduce the heat and let it simmer while it is partially covered until the volume is reduced to half the original volume.

3. Strain the mixture through a sieve or cheesecloth to remove the dill.

4. Measure 1 pint (500 mls) of the liquid and add the honey.

5. Cook for a few minutes as you stir it so that it thickens.

6. Store the syrup in an airtight container in the fridge for up to 2 months.

*****

Dill Poultice

Equipment

Cheesecloth or old cotton sheet strips

***

Ingredients

1 tablespoon bruised, fresh dill or powdered, dry dill

Boiling water

***

Instructions

1. Add enough boiling water to the dill to wet it and make a thick paste.

2. Spoon the dill paste onto the cheesecloth (or bed sheet strips) to make the poultice.

3. To use, apply the poultice to the affected area and cover with another piece of hot, wet cloth. Replace the hot, wet cloth when it cools with another hot one to keep the poultice hot.

*****

Dill Tincture

Equipment

Glass jar with tight fitting lid

Dark tincture bottles

Cheesecloth

Labels

***

Ingredients

7 oz (200 gm) of dried dill or 14 oz (400 gm) of fresh dill

30 oz (1 liter) of 80-100 proof vodka

***

Instructions

1. Fill 1/3 of the glass jar with the chopped dill.

2. Add the vodka to completely fill the jar to the top.

3. Seal the jar and label it with the date of preparation and name of dill used. Store the glass jar in a dark place for 6 weeks ensuring that you shake them weekly.

4. After 6 weeks strain out the dill with a cheesecloth and pour the tincture into dark tincture bottles.

5. Label the tincture bottles and store your herbal tinctures away from light and heat.

*****

Dill Infused Oil

Equipment

Double boiler

Large glass bowl

Sieve and cheesecloth

Sterilized dark jars

***

Ingredients

16 fl oz. (500 ml) vegetable oil like olive or sweet almond oil

8 oz. (250 grams) slightly crushed, dry dill or 16 oz. (500 grams) slightly bruised fresh dill

***

Instructions

1. Place the dill and oil in the glass bowl ensuring that the oil covers the dill. Simmer them in a double boiler for 1 hour at around 120 degrees Fahrenheit (49 degrees Celsius). Do not let the mixture boil. You can repeat this step after letting the oils cool to create more concentrated herb infused oils.

2. Strain the mixture through the sieve and cheesecloth into a clean, dark jar ensuring you squeeze out as much oil as you can from the cheesecloth.

3. Label your jars and store your dill infused oils in a cool dark place or in the refrigerator and use them within 3 months.

*****

Dill Butter

Equipment

Large glass bowl

Electric mixer or stick blender or wire whisk

Molds such as ice cube trays (optional)

***

Ingredients

½ cup butter

2 tablespoons of finely crushed, dried dill or 2 tablespoons of finely minced, fresh dill

***

Instructions

1. Place the butter in a warm place so that it can soften.

2. Put butter and dill in a large glass bowl and blend well until thoroughly mixed.

3. Refrigerate until it hardens. You can refrigerate it in molds or ice cube trays to give it a special shape.

*****

Dill Vinegar

Equipment

Large glass bottle with a well-fitting, non-metal lid or cork

***

Ingredients

1 pint (500 ml) white vinegar

2 tablespoons dill

***

Instructions

1. Place the dill in the glass bottle.

2. Add the vinegar and ensure that all the dill is covered by vinegar.

3. Seal the bottle and let it stand for up to 6 months. The longer it stands, the stronger the flavor becomes.

###

ABOUT THE AUTHOR

Marian Kim is an experienced alternative medicine practitioner.

OTHER BOOKS BY THE AUTHOR

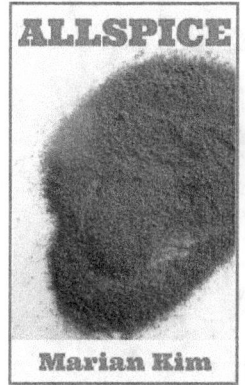

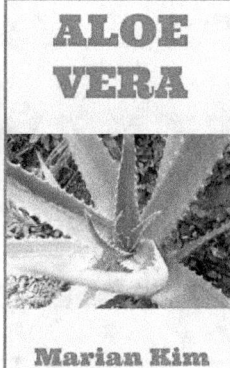

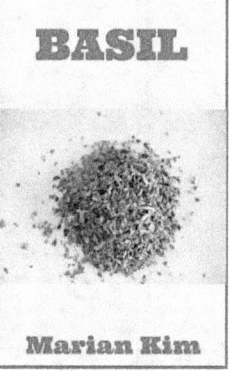

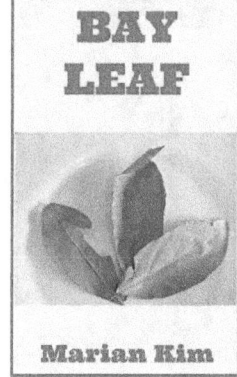

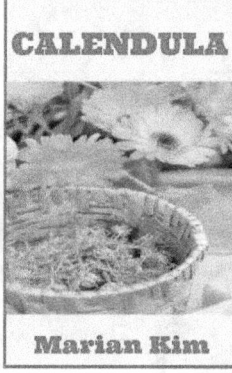

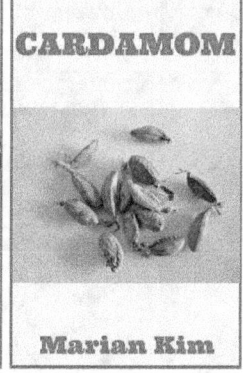

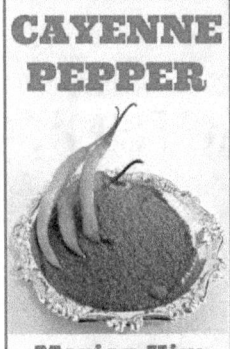

CAYENNE PEPPER

Marian Kim

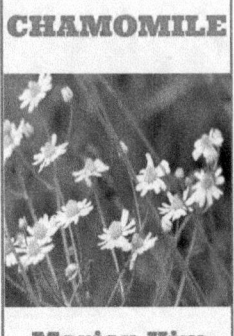

CHAMOMILE

Marian Kim

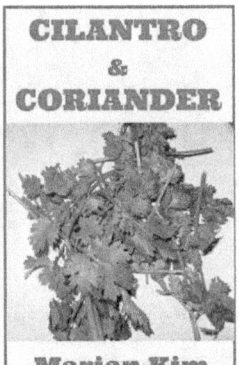

CILANTRO & CORIANDER

Marian Kim

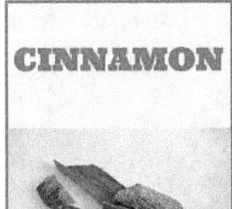

CINNAMON

Marian Kim

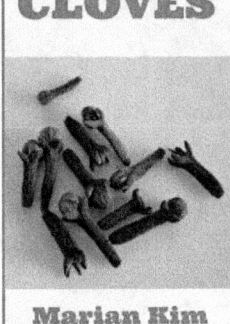

CLOVES

Marian Kim

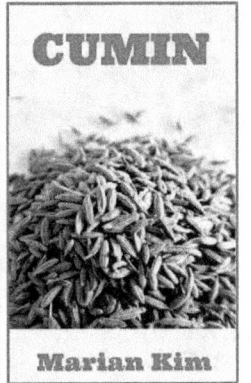

CUMIN

Marian Kim

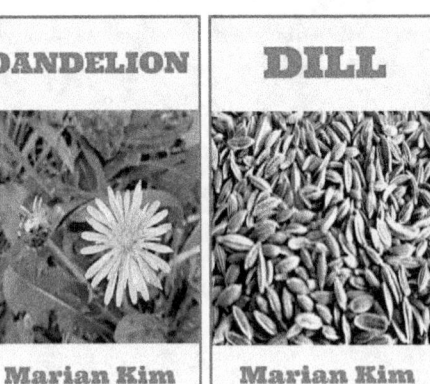

DANDELION

Marian Kim

DILL

Marian Kim

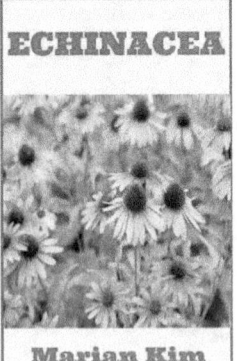

ECHINACEA

Marian Kim

FENNEL

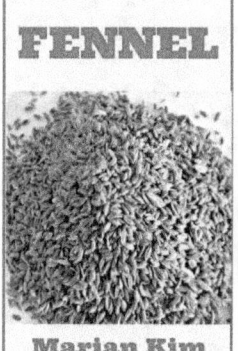

Marian Kim

FENUGREEK

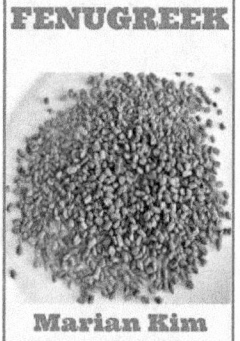

Marian Kim

GARLIC

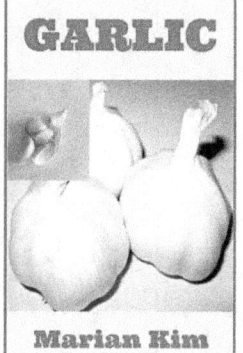

Marian Kim

GINGER

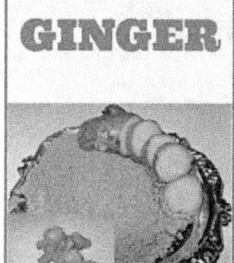

Marian Kim

GINKGO BILOBA

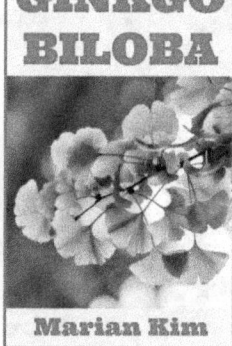

Marian Kim

GINSENG

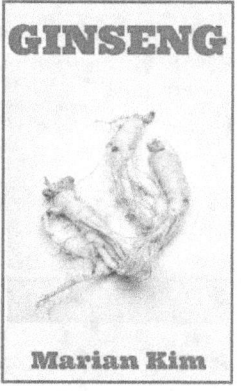

Marian Kim

LAVENDER

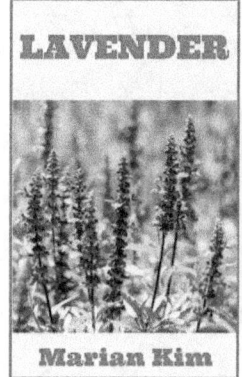

Marian Kim

MUSTARD

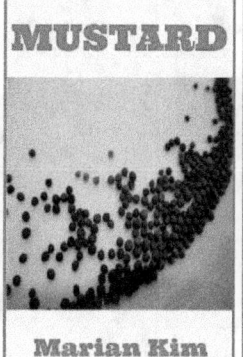

Marian Kim

NEEM

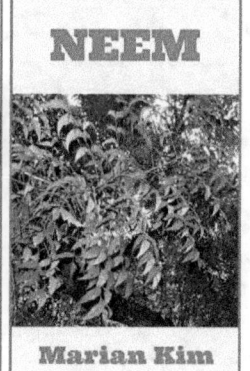

Marian Kim

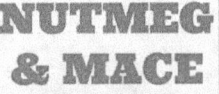

NUTMEG & MACE

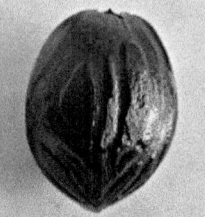

Marian Kim

OREGANO

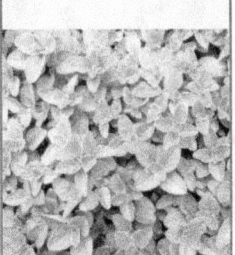

Marian Kim

PAPRIKA

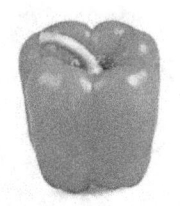

Marian Kim

PARSLEY

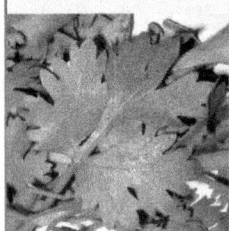

Marian Kim

BLACK & WHITE PEPPER

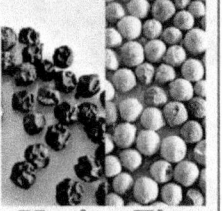

Marian Kim

PEPPERMINT

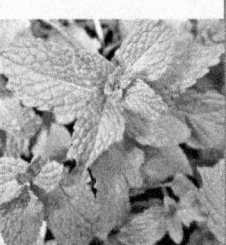

Marian Kim

ROSE HIPS

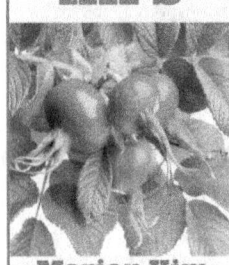

Marian Kim

ROSE PETALS

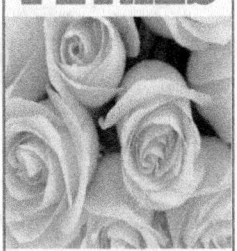

Marian Kim

ROSEMARY

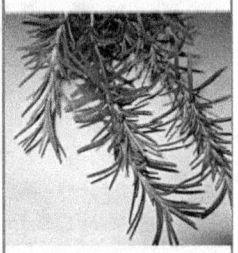

Marian Kim

SAGE

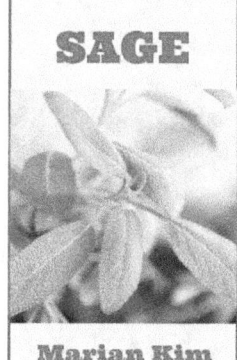

Marian Kim

ST. JOHN'S WORT

Marian Kim

STAR ANISE

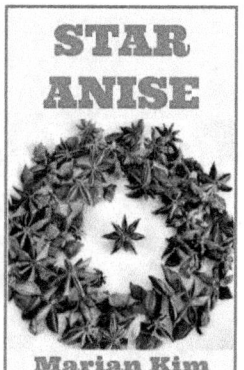

Marian Kim

STINGING NETTLE

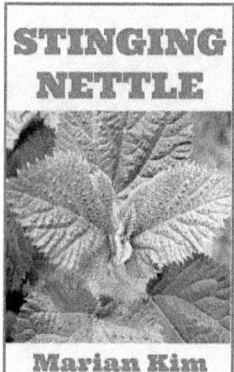

Marian Kim

THYME

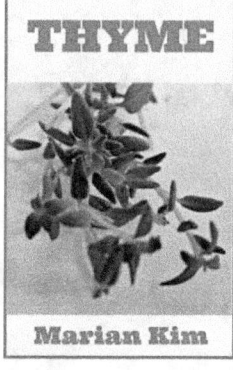

Marian Kim

TURMERIC

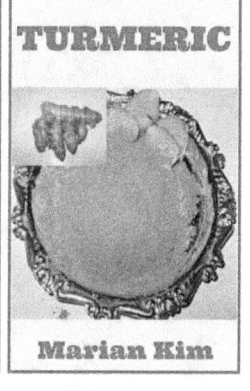

Marian Kim

WITCH HAZEL

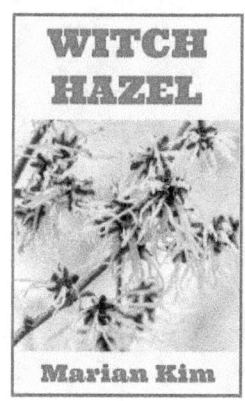

Marian Kim

YARROW

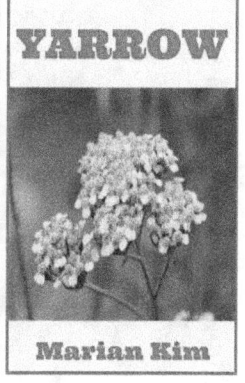

Marian Kim

*****